Principal Blood Disorders And Their Treatments

A practical guide to understanding and managing blood disorders

By Sylvia D. Robert

For permission requests, write to the copyright owner.

Table of contents

Chapter 1

Definition Of Blood

The human body's essential fluid, blood, travels throughout the circulatory system transporting waste products, nutrition, hormones, and oxygen. It is made up of platelets, plasma, and red and white blood cells.
A complicated biological fluid necessary for life support is blood. It makes up about 8% of the body weight and travels through blood arteries performing a number of vital tasks.

 Naturally, of course! There are a new key point to be aware of when discussing blood. Red blood cells, white blood cells, platelets, and plasma make up blood, to start.White blood cells aid in the body's defense against infection, whereas red blood cells transport oxygen throughout. Platelets aid in blood clotting and stop bleeding. All of these components are transported throughout the body by plasma. Additionally, blood has a wide range of proteins and enzymes that support several bodily processes. It is an intricate and essential bodily component.

The body's blood is an intricate and essential component. It is composed of numerous distinct parts, each of which has a distinct function. The fluid that contains everything is called plasma. Red blood cells deliver oxygen, white blood cells fight infection, and platelets aid in clotting. A range of proteins and enzymes can also be found in blood. Together, these elements support the body's normal operation.

Chapter 2

Definition Of Blood Diseases and Causes

Blood Disease:
Hematologic diseases, sometimes referred to as blood diseases, are conditions that impact the blood and organs that create blood, such as the spleen or bone marrow. Numerous reasons, including genetics, infections, or other medical disorders, can be the cause. Anemia, leukemia, lymphoma, sickle cell disease, and thrombocytopenia are examples of common blood disorders. While some blood disorders

are benign and treatable, others may be extremely dangerous and even fatal.

There are numerous varieties of blood illnesses, which means there are numerous possible causes. Blood diseases can arise from a variety of common causes, such as immune system abnormalities, infections, hereditary factors, and specific drugs. Toxin exposure is one of the environmental variables that can also cause some blood illnesses. For more precise information, it's important to speak with a physician or other medical professional as there are numerous other potential causes. Additional potential reasons for blood abnormalities include malnourishment, radiation exposure, specific malignancies, specific autoimmune conditions, and specific congenital conditions.

Blood diseases can also be caused by a wide range of uncommon conditions, including certain metabolic diseases and hereditary abnormalities. As you can see, blood illnesses can have a wide range of intricate causes. Because of this, it's crucial that you consult a medical expert if you have any worries about your health.

Chapter 3

Blood Conditions

Introduction: Anemia is defined as a reduction in the amount of hemoglobin present in red blood cells. This lecture will lead to the classification of anemia into two main categories: anatomical classification and physiological classification.

Anaemia's Physical Classification and Causes It is not the form or color of the red blood cell that causes this, but rather its aberrant function. tion.

The precise definition of anemia is a reduction in red blood cell (RBC) mass. Delivering oxygen from the lungs to the tissues and carbon dioxide from the tissues to the lungs is the role of the red blood cell. The process makes use of hemoglobin (Hb). Anemia is characterized by a reduction of red blood cells

(RBCs) that carry oxygen and carbon dioxide, which hinders the body's ability to exchange glasses. REDuced RBC synthesis, increased hemolysis (the breakdown of red blood cells), or blood loss could be the cause of the decline.hemoglobin deficiency. Iron deficiency in the body is the primary cause of this most prevalent kind of anemia.

Iron is needed by your bone marrow to produce hemoglobin. Your body cannot create enough hemoglobin for red blood cells if you don't consume enough iron.

Many pregnant women experience this kind of anemia if they do not take iron supplements. Blood loss from heavy menstrual bleeding, ulcers, and frequent use of some over-the-counter painkillers—particularly aspirin, which can induce inflammation of the stomach lining and result in blood loss—are other causes of it.

Anemia caused by a lack of vitamins {pernicious anemia}. Besides iron, your body needs vitamin B-12 to produce healthy red blood cells. A diet lacking in these and other key nutrients can cause decreased red blood cell production.

Furthermore, some individuals who have B-12 don't absorb the vitamin. Pernicious anemia, another name for vitamin-deficient anemia, may result from this.

Anaplastic syndrome. Anemia is an uncommon and potentially fatal condition caused by insufficient production of red blood cells in the body. Aplastic anemia can be brought on by exposure to hazardous chemicals, autoimmune disorders, infections, and specific medications. Many illnesses, including leukemia and myelofibrosis, can impact your bone marrow's ability to produce blood, which can result in anemia. These cancers and cancer-like illnesses can have mild to potentially fatal consequences. A few illnesses, including kidney disease, rheumatoid arthritis, cancer, HIV/AIDS,red blood cell production can also be hampered by Crohn's disease and other acute or chronic inflammatory illnesses.

hemolytic anemia. When red blood cells are lost more quickly than the bone marrow can produce new ones, anemia in this category develops. Red blood cell degeneration is accelerated by certain blood disorders. Hemolytic anemia can be inherited or acquired later in life. The condition linked to RBCs having a shorter lifespan is called hemolytic anemia.

RBCs' reduced lifespan could be caused by an extracorpuscular or intracorpuscular anomaly. The rate of destruction and the elimination of RBCs determine the severity.

The anemia might not become noticeable until the RBCs have only 20 days left in their lifespan because a healthy bone marrow can increase its workload by 6 to 8 times.Hemolytic anemia causes:Hereditary intrinsic abnormalities, such as abnormal RBC membrane deficiencies and spherocytosis, are inherited.genetic disorders affecting the RBCs, such as G-6-phosphate dehydrogenase deficiency.abnormalities in the manufacturing of hemoglobin, such as sickle cell disease.syndrome of thalassemia.hemoglobinuria, nocturnal paroxysmal.Chemical and poisonous agents are examples of extrinsic defects.Hemolysis is brought on by infection.Hypersplenism.hemolytic anemia immune.sickle cell disease. Hemolytic anemia is a genetic disorder that can occasionally be rather dangerous. The aberrant crescent (sickle) shape of red blood cells is caused by a faulty type of hemoglobin.

There is a persistent lack of red blood cells as a result of these abnormal blood cells dying too soon.

Megaloblastic Anaemia: A compromised DNA synthesis is the cause of megaloblastic anemia. The most common causes of megaloblastic anemia are folic acid and vitamin B12 deficiencies.

One might categorize megaloblastic anemia into:

Anemia brought on by a vitamin B12 deficiency.

Anemia brought on by a folic acid deficit.

The third group is not responsive to folic acid or vitamin B12 therapy.

Megaloblastic anemia can be caused by deficiencies in vitamin B12.

a lack of folic acid. Its inadequacy has numerous causes. The majority of them have dietary roots.

The body stores folic acid for only three months. When demand is high, it can result in deficiency, pregnancy, rapid growth in infancy and adolescence, poor folate intake, and

alcoholism. Malabsorption syndrome can cause folic acid deficiency, which can be inhibited by medications such as birth control pills and anticonvulsant drugs. Erythroid hyperplasia is seen in the bone marrow. EYES: yellowing; SKIN: paleness, yellowing, and coldness of hands and feet; RESPIRATORY: shortness of breath; MUSCULAR: weakness; Internal: change in stool color; CNS: fatigue, dizziness, and fainting; BLOOD VESSELS: low blood pressure
Heart: angina, chest pain, palpitations, fast heartbeat, and heart attack
SPLEEN enlargement.

ANATOMY AND MORPHOLOGY OF RED BLOOD CELLS
Anemia normochromic and normocytic:
Red blood cells stained normally with a central pallor are referred to as normochromic. Normocytic also describes normal red blood cells, which have a diameter of 8 μm.
Results from the lab:
low level of hemoglobin.

80 to 95 fL is the normal mean corpuscular volume (MCV).

The mean corpuscular hemoglobin (MCH) should be at least 27 pg.

normal mean concentration of hemoglobin in corpuscles. (MCHC)

These are mostly brought on by sudden blood loss.

N/B: Normal red blood cell morphology is typified by a donut-shaped red blood cell with a pale or hemoglobin-free central third. The peripheral smear is used to evaluate this.

Microcytic and hypochromic anemia

Red blood cells that stain pale and have a large area of central pallor are referred to as such.

The reasons are:

This is brought on by an iron deficit, which is caused by a decrease in dietary iron intake or poor absorption.

hemoglobin deficiency.

poisoned with lead.

thalassemia.

Prolonged bleeding may result in an increased loss of iron.

An irregularity in iron metabolism could exist.
The body's increased need throughout infancy.
pregnancy and nursing.
because of cancer.
bleeding disorders.
Hookworms.
medication such as salicylates (aspirin).
Results from the lab:
Males <12 g/dL and females <10 g/dL have low
hemoglobin levels.PCV<30%
Minimal MCV of less than 80 fL.
MCH less than 27 pages.
Pale, hypochromic RBCs and microcytes are
visible in peripheral blood smears.
A leucopenia may be present.
In the event of bleeding, platelets are high.
Reticulocyte counts are lower than anticipated
due to anemia.
Erythroid hyperplasia is seen in the bone
marrow.
Very low iron is shown by iron stains.
HYPERCHROMIC
IC MACROCYTIC ANAEMIA:
This describes red blood cells that are larger
than usual, have a diameter larger than 8 µm,
an immature nucleus, and exhibit excessive red

staining with diminished central pallor.For example, leukemia, intrinsic factor deficiency, and megaloblastic anemia.

Results from the lab:

Low MCV > 99 fL; hemoglobin < 10 g/dl.

The peripheral blood smear displays many hypersegmentation of neutrophils as well as macrocytosis.

I occasionally see thrombocytopenia and leukopenia.

The reasons are:

Folic acid reserve are only good for three months.

Increased demand can result in deficiencies such as pregnancy, early childhood growth, and puberty.

in cases of fast transitions such as drunkenness, hemolytic anemia, and inadequate folate intake.

Malabsorption syndrome can result in folic acid insufficiency, which can be exacerbated by medications such as anticonvulsants and birth control tablets.

Deficiency in Vitamin B12

The cause of megaloblastic anemia is faulty DNA synthesis.

There are two categories of megaloblastic anemia: i. anemia resulting from a vitamin B12 deficiency.
ii. Folic acid deficiency-related anemia
iii. Neither folic acid for vitamin B12 therapy has any effect on the third group.

Treatments for anemia
The underlying cause of anemia determines how to treat it. Common treatments include iron supplements, vitamin B12 injections, diet modifications, and taking care of any underlying conditions, including chronic illnesses or gastrointestinal bleeding. For individualized guidance depending on the particular type and cause of anemia, speak with a healthcare professional.
vider.

Chapter 4

Leukemia
What is leukemia?
One kind of cancer that affects the bone marrow and blood is called leukemia. White

blood cells, which are in charge of battling infection, are growing abnormally in this situation. There are four basic forms of leukemia: acute myeloid leukemia (AML), acute lymphoblastic leukemia (ALL), chronic lymphocytic leukemia (CLL), and chronic myeloid leukemia (CML). Leukemia can be acute or chronic. Fatigue, easy bleeding or bruising, recurrent infections, and weight loss are possible symptoms. Treatment options for leukemia vary according to its type and stage and can include stem cell transplantation, radiation therapy, and chemotherapy.

 A qualified healthcare provider must be consulted in order to receive an accurate diagnosis and treatment plan.

Leukemia can have many different causes, but the three most prevalent ones are viruses, environmental factors, and genetics. Leukemia risk, for instance, may rise in response to specific inherited genetic abnormalities. Environmental elements that can raise the risk include exposure to radiation and certain chemicals. Furthermore, some viruses—like the human T-cell leukemia virus—have been connected to the emergence of specific leukemia subtypes. Aplastic anemia and myelodysplastic syndromes are two more underlying illnesses that can occasionally lead to leukemia. Leukemia has numerous risk factors, however some of the most prevalent ones are age, family history, exposure to chemicals or radiation, as well as a few other medical issues. The incidence of leukemia is higher in older persons and in those with a family history of the illness. Leukemia risk can also be increased by radiation exposure from medical operations or nuclear accidents. Leukemia has also been connected to certain chemicals, including vinyl chloride and benzene. Leukemia cases can have a variety of causes, and other additional risk factors.

Solutions

Treatment for Leukemia

Instead of using natural cures, modern methods are usually used to treat leukemia. Typical therapeutic choices consist of:

Chemotherapy: drugs used to either eradicate or inhibit the growth of cancer cells.
High-dose X-rays or other high-energy radiation are used in radiation treatment to kill cancer cells.
Stem cell transplantation: using healthy stem cells to replace defective or damaged bone marrow
Drugs known as "targeted therapy" aim to minimize harm to healthy cells by selectively attacking cancer cells.
Immunotherapy: enhancing the immune system to aid in the battle against cancer
Healthcare providers and oncologists frequently oversee the administration of these treatments. Those who have been diagnosed with leukemia should speak with their medical team to figure out the best course of action for their particular type and stage of the disease.
ase.

Chapter 5

Lymphoma

A kind of blood cancer called lymphoma originates in the body's lymphatic system, which is a component of the immune system. Although there are many distinct varieties of lymphomas, all of them are malignancies that start in the lymphatic system, so the name "lymphoma" is fairly general. Hodgkin lymphoma and non-Hodgkin lymphoma are the two primary forms of lymphoma. Although disease can strike anyone at any age, persons over 50 are more likely to get lymphoma.

The type and intensity of lymphoma can affect the symptoms that a patient experiences. Swollen lymph nodes, fever, sweats at night, exhaustion, weight loss, and itching are typical symptoms. More severe symptoms, such as breathing difficulties, swallowing difficulties, or bone pain, may also be present in rare cases. Get a proper diagnosis from a doctor because a lot of these symptoms might be caused by other ailments.

Solutions:

Chemotherapy, a kind of medication therapy that destroys cancer cells, is the primary treatment for many forms of lymphoma. Stem cell transplantation and immunotherapy are further potential treatments that harness the body's immune system to combat cancer. Certain patients may also benefit from radiation therapy, surgery, or targeted therapy, depending on the kind and stage of their lymphoma.

Chapter 6

Hemophilia

The hereditary bleeding disorder hemophilia impairs the body's capacity to coagulate blood. Individuals with hemophilia bleed after an injury for longer than usual because they lack a protein called clotting factor. Hemophilia A and B are the two primary forms of hemophilia. The most prevalent kind, hemophilia A, is brought on by a lack of clotting factor VIII. Clotting factor IX deficiency is the cause of hemophilia B. One can have mild, moderate, or severe forms of both.

Hemophilia is a subject that has many more facets. It's important to realize that bleeding can occur both internally and externally in hemophiliacs. Internal bleeding can happen in the brain, muscles, or joints, and it can be quite serious.

External bleeding happens at the site of an injury and is more frequent. Hemophiliacs must take clotting factor medication in order to control bleeding and avoid problems. The therapy is frequently administered at home via intravenous means. Anemia and joint degeneration are among the additional health issues that some hemophiliacs may experience.

Solutions

Hemophilia can be treated with a variety of methods. Giving the patient the missing clotting factor is known as replacement treatment, and it is the most used type of car. Infusions or injections can be used for this. Additionally, there are medications that can increase the body's production of clotting factors. Surgery could be required in some circumstances to fix broken joints or other tissues. Physical therapy can help some hemophiliacs with their condition by increasing joint mobility and function. Yes, desmopressin is another treatment option for hemophilia. This hormone aids in the body's removal of clotting components that have accumulated in blood vessels. Desmopressin may not be appropriate for everyone and is usually reserved for mild cases of hemophilia. It's crucial to discuss all of the available treatment choices with a doctor and determine which is best for your particular situation.

Chapter 7

Thrombocytopenia

A person with thrombocytopenia has insufficient platelets, which are blood cells that aid in blood clotting. Thrombocytopenia can be brought on by a variety of factors, such as genetic illnesses, autoimmune diseases, and certain drugs. It might also result from cancer therapy adverse effects. Serious bleeding, even potentially fatal hemorrhage, can be brought on by thrombocytopenia.

A platelet count of less than 150,000 per microliter (µL) of blood is another definition of thrombocytopenia. Bleeding risk can be elevated by a low platelet count since platelets are tiny cells that aid in blood clotting. Thrombocytopenia can be classified into two basic types: primary thrombocytopenia, which is caused by a bone marrow deficiency, and secondary thrombocytopenia, which is caused by another disease or condition.

The most typical sign of thrombocytopenia is easy bruising or bleeding, which manifests as bleeding gums or red or purple areas on the skin.

Blood in the urine or stool, severe menstrual bleeding, nosebleeds, and excessive bleeding from injuries are some other signs. It's critical to consult a physician immediately if you have any of these symptoms. Depending on the underlying reason, thrombocytopenia can have a wide range of therapies.

Solutions

Depending on the underlying reason, treatment for thrombocytopenia may involve platelet transfusions, treating the underlying illness, administering corticosteroids or immunoglobulins, or taking drugs to boost platelet production.

The most popular therapies include steroids, blood transfusions, and drugs that increase the synthesis of platelets.The spleen, an organ that aids in blood filtering, may also need to be surgically removed in certain cases of thrombocytopenia. Treating the underlying illness, such as cancer or an infection, may also assist to raise the platelet count if thrombocytopenia is the result of it.

 A medical professional's advice is essential for obtaining a precise diagnosis and a suitable treatment strategy.

Chapter 8

Sickle Cell Illness

Hemoglobin, the protein that delivers oxygen in red blood cells, is faulty in sickle cell disease (SCD), an inherited blood illness. Certain situations cause hemoglobin in people with sickle cell disease (SCD) to develop a "sickle" shape, which can cause a number of difficulties.

Pain Crises: Because the malformed red blood cells obstruct blood flow, sickle cell disease (SCD) results in painful episodes known as pain crises.

Anemia: Because sickle cells live shorter lives, there is a persistent deficiency of red blood cells, which causes anemia.

Organ Damage: As the spleen, liver, and kidneys attempt to filter out and process the aberrant cells, the changed cells might cause harm to these organs and tissues.

Infections: Because the spleen is a key organ in the immune system, it may not work as well in people with sickle cell disease (SCD), making them more vulnerable to infections.

Stroke: SCD, especially in young patients, may raise the risk of stroke.

Similar to pneumonia, acute chest syndrome is a dangerous condition involving inflammation of the lungs.

Supportive treatment is part of the SCD management process; it helps to reduce symptoms and avoid complications. This comprises:blood transfusions, pain treatment, and, in extreme circumstances, bone marrow or stem cell transplants. Maintaining a healthy lifestyle that includes staying hydrated and avoiding triggers, along with routine medical checkups, are crucial for controlling the illness. People with sickle cell disease can live far better lives if they receive comprehensive care and an early diagnosis.

Solutions

Even though sickle cell disease has no known cure, there are a number of interventions and therapies that can help control symptoms and enhance quality of life:

Pain Control: One important feature of SCD is the occurrence of pain crises. Prescription or over-the-counter painkillers may be used for pain treatment.

Hydration: Maintaining adequate hydration helps stop sickle cell adhesion and blood vessel obstructions.

Blood Transfusions: Transfusions can enhance oxygen flow and boost the quantity of healthy red blood cells.

Hydroxyurea: This drug can increase the fetal hemoglobin ability to withstand sickness.

Stem cell or bone marrow transplant: In extreme circumstances, a transplant from a suitable donor can be taken into consideration as a possible treatment.

Antibiotics: Due to the higher susceptibility of people with sickle cell disease (SCD), prophylactic antibiotics are frequently provided to avoid infection.
Vaccinations: Vaccinations are a preventive measure against illnesses, which can be especially risky for people with weakened immune systems.

Pulmonary Care: Oxygen therapy or other forms of respiratory support may be necessary for the management of lung problems, such as acute chest syndrome.

Frequent medical examinations: Early detection and management of problems can lead to better results. It's crucial to see healthcare professionals on a regular basis

Chapter 9

The polycythemia

 An excessive number of red blood cells in the blood is known as polycythemia. This may result in thickening and sluggish blood flow, which may produce a number of symptoms such as headaches, dizziness, dyspnea, and a fast heart rate.

Primary polycythemia and secondary polycythemia are the two main forms of polycythemia. Whereas secondary polycythemia is brought on by an additional underlying illness, such as heart or lung disease, primary polycythemia is brought on by a problem with the bone marrow. A feeling of fullness in the left upper abdomen (due to an enlarged spleen) is one of the symptoms of polycythemia, in addition to the previously listed ones. Other symptoms include blurred or double vision, easy bruising or bleeding, and a variety of skin changes, including rashes, itching, and redness.

Polycythemia can potentially lead to some very significant side effects, such as stroke, heart failure, and blood clots. Those who have secondary polycythemia are more likely to have problems.

Let's now discuss polycythemia's causes. A mutation in the JAK2 gene can result in primary polycythemia by causing the bone marrow to create an excessive amount of red blood cells. Numerous other disorders can also lead to secondary polycythemia, such as pulmonary hypertension, hypoxia (low oxygen levels), obstructive sleep apnea, high altitude, high levels of certain hormones (such as erythropoietin), kidney, liver, and cardiac problems.

Primary polycythemia and secondary polycythemia are the two main forms of polycythemia. Whereas secondary polycythemia is brought on by an additional underlying illness, such as heart or lung disease, primary polycythemia is brought on by a problem with the bone marrow.A feeling of fullness in the left upper abdomen (due to an enlarged spleen) is one of the symptoms of polycythemia, in addition to the previously listed ones. Other symptoms include blurred or double vision, easy bruising or bleeding, and a variety of skin changes, including rashes, itching, and redness.

After discussing the signs and causes of polycythemia, I'd like to move on to the topic of diagnosis and prevention. A physician will do a physical examination and obtain a medical history in order to diagnose polycythemia. Additionally, they can request blood tests, such as a complete blood count (CBC), which might reveal anomalies and high red blood cell counts. A bone marrow biopsy, which might reveal alterations in the bone marrow, is one of the additional procedures that might be performed. Let's go on to prevention. The best defense against polycythemia is to treat any underlying illnesses, such as hypoxia or sleep apnea.

Solutions

Now, let's begin with phlebotomy, which is the primary treatment for polycythemia.
Through the removal of blood from the body, the red blood cell count is lowered during this treatment. Medication may be recommended in addition to phlebotomy to address the underlying cause of polycythemia. Aspirin, which can help avoid blood clots, and hydroxyurea, which lowers the red blood cell count, are two examples of these drugs. Diuretics, oxygen therapy, and lifestyle modifications such as avoiding high-altitude settings are possible further treatments.

Chapter 10

HIV/AIDS
The human immunodeficiency virus, or HIV,is a blood illness that can impair immunity and lead to HIV/AIDS (illness of the immune system)
Blood is one physiological fluid through which

HIV can spread, and if treatment is not received, the virus can be fatal. Nonetheless, people with HIV can now live long, healthy lives because of advancements in treatment. In order to manage HIV and stop it from developing into AIDS, early diagnosis and treatment are essential.

HIV can spread and result in AIDS in a number of ways. even if they are less widespread. One way is through unintentional needles, such as when a medical professional pokes themselves with a needle that has been used in a patient who is HIV positive.

Another method involves coming into contact with contaminated blood, such as from a cut or wound that gets infected. HIV can potentially be acquired by organ transplantation from an infected donor, although this is extremely uncommon.

The most popular method is having unprotected intercourse with an HIV-positive person. Other methods include getting an infected blood transfusion, exchanging syringes or needles with an infected individual, or being born to an HIV-positive mother. Furthermore, those with compromised immune systems are more vulnerable to HIV infection. This encompasses both individuals who have undergone organ transplantation and those who suffer from other illnesses like cancer.

Apart from the previously stated methods, transfer from mother to child can also result in HIV infection. This happens when a mother who is HIV positive transmits the virus to her unborn child during pregnancy, childbirth, or breastfeeding. Although it is less common, oral sex can potentially spread HIV. Saliva, sweat, and tears are not prevalent ways of HIV transmission, while there are extremely rare reports of it happening. It is imperative to comprehend all the modes of HIV transmission in order to implement appropriate preventive measures.

Solutions:

Various therapy modalities are available for HIV, contingent on the disease's stage and additional variables. Treatment with antiretroviral therapy (ART) is the most prevalent.

It employs a mix of drugs to lower the body's HIV concentration and delay the disease's progression. Post-exposure prophylaxis (PEP), which is taking antiretroviral medication as soon as possible after HIV exposure, is an additional therapeutic option. PEP has the ability to stop the virus from infecting the body and taking hold.

Chapter 11

General Treatments for Blood Diseases
Nutrition and diet:
For blood health as well as general health, a balanced diet is essential. Red meat, chicken, fish, leafy greens, legumes, and fortified cereals are a few foods high in iron. Rich sources of vitamin B12 include seafood, poultry, chicken, and dairy products. Citrus fruits, legumes, and leafy greens are foods high in folic acid.

Drinking lots of water will help you stay hydrated in addition to eating a balanced diet. Lastly, excessive alcohol intake should be avoided, as it may have a bad effect on blood health.

Let's now discuss the relationship between preventing blood problems and maintaining a healthy diet. Iron deficiency anemia and vitamin B12 deficiency are two blood disorders that are less likely to develop with a healthy diet. Eating a diet high in iron can prevent iron deficiency anemia, while eating a diet high in vitamin B12 can prevent vitamin B12 deficiency.

A nutritious diet can also help lower the risk of leukemia and other cancers that can affect the blood.

Changes in lifestyle

Making changes to one's lifestyle might be just as crucial to blood health maintenance as dietary changes. Frequent exercise can lower the risk of blood disorders, including blood clots, and enhance cardiovascular health. In addition to lowering inflammation, stress management can improve general health. Additionally, keeping a strong immune system, which in turn supports blood health, depends on obtaining enough sleep. Thus, it's critical to ensure that you exercise on a regular basis,controlling your stress and obtaining enough rest to maintain the health of your blood.

Let's now discuss some particular lifestyle changes that can help maintain blood health. For instance, aerobic and weight training should both be a part of a regular exercise regimen. Exercises that promote cardiovascular fitness, such as jogging or brisk walking, also help to develop muscle and improve bone density. Meditating or deep breathing are examples of relaxation techniques that can be used in stress management. Additionally, 7-9 hours of sleep per night are necessary to achieve adequate sleep.

I would also like to emphasize that quitting smoking is essential for maintaining healthy blood.

Anemia, heart disease, blood clots, and other blood disorders are all significantly increased by smoking. Thus, it's critical to develop a plan to stop smoking as soon as possible if you currently smoke. Recall that leading a healthy

lifestyle can significantly affect your blood health, so continue on your current path!
Alternative Medical Interventions
To support blood health, a variety of complementary and alternative therapies can be employed in addition to conventional treatments. For instance, acupuncture is a kind of traditional Chinese medicine in which tiny needles are inserted into certain body spots in order to help regulate energy flow and encourage healing. Astragalus and ginseng are two examples of herbal medicines that might boost immunity and lesen inflammation. Additionally, mindfulness exercises like yoga or meditation can support relaxation and help people feel less stressed.
Yoga is a mind-body discipline that incorporates breathing techniques, physical postures, and meditation. Yoga can benefit both mental and physical well-being. No matter your age, experience level, or degree of fitness, yoga is for you. Yoga is a journey rather than a goal; improvement is attained with practice.
It's crucial to keep in mind that while therapies can be used in addition to conventional medical care to support general health and wellness,

they shouldn't be utilized in place of it. Consult your physician to see whether any of these treatments are a good fit for you.

Support Groups and Mental Health: Stress, anxiety, and sadness are common side effects of blood illnesses that can have a negative impact on a person's mental health. People can find a secure place to talk about their feelings and experiences with others who are sympathetic to what they're going through in support groups. Dealing with the psychological difficulties of having a blood disorder can also be helped by counseling or therapy. It's critical to keep in mind that asking for assistance is acceptable and that the tools are accessible to promote mental wellness.

Individuals impacted by blood disorders can join any of the many support groups provided by the American Red Cross. Along with support groups and resources, other national organizations also exist, including the Leukemia and Lymphoma Society,the National Marrow

Donor Program and the American Cancer Society.

Treatment Innovations: In recent years, where have been a number of fascinating developments in the management of blood disorders. The emergence of gene therapy, which employs altered genes to treat or prevent certain blood disorders, is one instance. Additionally, novel drugs are being created, such as targeted medicines for the treatment of blood disorders including lymphoma and leukemia. Nowadays, stem cell transplants are among the safer and more effective treatments available.

The creation of CAR T-cell therapy is among the most revolutionary advancements in medical science. This kind of immunotherapy targets and destroys cancer cells by using genetically altered T-cells, a subset of white blood cells. CAR T-cell treatment is currently being researched for various blood disorders and has demonstrated efficacy in treating certain forms of lymphoma and leukemia.

Remark: In CAR T-cell treatment, a patient's T cells are extracted and subsequently altered genetically in a laboratory. After being reinjected into the patient's body, the altered T-cells hunt out and destroy cancer cells. Each patient receives a customized course of treatment, which is now being researched for a number of blood disorders. Although CAR T-cell therapy is still a relatively new medicine, early results from clinical trials indicate great promise.

Preventive Measures: Keeping your blood healthy starts with taking preventive measures. Regular check-ups, which include blood testing, can aid in the early detection of any possible issues.

Vaccinating against some diseases, like human papillomavirus (HPV) and hepatitis B, can also lower the chance of getting several blood problems. Additionally, spreading knowledge about the value of routine medical exams and early identification can aid in the prevention of

the onset or worsening of many blood disorders.
World Blood Donor Day is one initiative that has significantly improved blood health. This yearly event, which takes place on June 14th, strives to emphasize the value of blood donation and increase awareness of how donors can save lives. Worldwide blood donations have increased as a result of this campaign, which has also saved many lives.

Chapter 12

In brief:
"Principal Blood Disorders and Their Treatments" explorer the complexities of different blood illnesses, providing a thorough analysis of their symptoms, causes, and traditional treatments. The book covers disorders like anemia, leukemia, hemophilia, and thrombosis, giving readers a good understanding of the effects these illnesses have on people's lives. It carefully describes the scientific underpinnings of every illness, making it readable by readers who are not medical professionals.

The section on remedies provides a useful manual that explains dietary modifications, lifestyle changes, and traditional medical measures that can be used to control or lessen the symptoms of various blood illnesses.
By combining technical medical knowledge with approachable language, the book gives readers the information they need to make wise decisions about their health.

Conclusion:
"Principal Blood Disorders and Their Treatments" emphasizes the value of holistic health care in the last few chapters. It promotes a multifaceted strategy that includes continual therapy advancements, lifestyle modifications, emotional support, and medicinal interventions. By promoting proactive participation in one's health and cultivating optimism for the future through emerging medical discoveries, the book leaves readers feeling empowered. In the end, it is an invaluable tool for people looking

for a thorough grasp of blood disorders and useful tactics for their health.

"Principal Blood Disorders and Their Treatments" explorer the complexities of different blood illnesses, providing a thorough analysis of their symptoms, causes, and traditional treatments. The book covers disorders like anemia, leukemia, hemophilia, and thrombosis, giving readers a good understanding of the effects these illnesses have on people's lives. It carefully describes the scientific underpinnings of every illness, making it readable by readers who are not medical professionals.

The section on remedies provides a useful manual that explains dietary modifications, lifestyle changes, and traditional medical measures that can be used to control or lessen the symptoms of various blood illnesses.